NEGATIVE CALORIE DIET

Lose Up To 10 Pounds a Week and Improve Your Health and Energy (Negative Calorie Diet Book Series)

By JESSICA RENEAU

Table of Contents

Copyright Notice

Disclaimer

Introduction

I believe that you have already heard about the magical food with so- called "negative calories" and quite reasonably you are wondering how can it be possible that any food has negative calories? The only food, if we count it as food, that has zero calories is water. Therefore, you are right, there isn't any other kind of food with zero or negative calorie amount, but nevertheless some food can act in that way because they contain less calories than your body really needs to transform into pure energy, so it could work properly. In this book, you will find many answers on how to "force" your body to start using its own reserves that it holds in the form of fatty tissue and how this specific food will boost your metabolism to work faster and to burn your fat reserve.

You shouldn't mix up terms "negative calorie food" and "empty calories" that are found in processed food or as most of us call it "junk food". If you think that this diet allows you to eat junk food then it's much better to quit reading it right now, but if you want to learn what kind of food belongs to the so called Negative calorie diet, then this book presents one of the best sources, where you will find many answers, tips and some meal proposals that will help you stick to this diet.

Chapter 1: Benefits of Negative calorie diet

To understand negative caloric diet first you need to understand some basic things related to nutrition. The basic knowledge includes answers about what are terms as: metabolism, basal metabolism and digestion. Whenever we eat or drink something, it means that we provide a "fuel" for our basic function as breathing, initiating of our muscle and nervous system to work. The main catch is that we often consume more food or to be specific more calories than our body really need and that excess is stored in our fatty tissue. Also, we all know that the basic of every kind of food consist from carbohydrates, fats and proteins, and the main difference is in the ratio of those nutrients in type of food that we eat.

When we say **digestion** it means every action that our body makes to break down the food into smaller simplified forms (carbohydrates mainly into glucose, fats into long-chain fatty acids and proteins into amino acids). All waste that's left after digestion, expellees through colon in form of feces. So, digestion starts from mouth and ends with poop.

Metabolism on the other hand is a chemical process in which nutrients are used as a fuel, mostly from glucose molecules, but this isn't the only source of energy, because when it comes to lack of carbs (specifically glucose), then fatty tissue present the main source of energy, because our brain send signal that our body is in "starvation mode" and fats become the main source of energy that is needed for normal function or **basal metabolism**. The basal metabolism therefore presents the minimum amount of energy with which our body needs to sustain first of all the body temperature and then all other processes in our body (cell regeneration, breathing process and so on).

When we use term "calories" it presents just a tool for measuring energy in our body and the term fatty tissue implies energy in form of all fats that is stored as a reserve in our organism.

When you enter the so- called negative caloric food it means that you enter food with lower caloric amount then our body needs for successful breakdown. Because our body needs more energy it starts to use stored energy, so it could be capable of finishing digestion and all metabolism processes. Unfortunately, this diet doesn't differ from any restrictive diet when it comes to whole day calorie intake that you may enter, but the good thing is that it includes many kinds of food that are very low in calories in ratio of the quantity of food that you may enter during a day.

The first benefit is that with this diet, you will control your feeling of hunger and so take over the control of your appetite, because your plate will be full with food all the time. The "negative caloric food" mostly presents food rich in fibers and low in simple sugar so it acts almost as a natural laxative and it will remove all excess of water from your body. It will also, help your guts work "harder "so it influences on accelerate digestion too. The best part is that if you suffer from higher cholesterol and triglycerides level in your bloodstream with "negative caloric food" you will lower them to health-safe level in a very short time. Negative caloric food is mostly used in detoxification process so you will preserve not only your blood vessels, but also your liver and kidneys (they are after all the main weapon against harmful substances that we enter into our body, not only with food but also through air we are breathing, or through skin when we shower).

This diet will after all keep you in a better shape, provide more beneficial antioxidants and definitely relive your body from many harmful free radicals, so overall it will get your health condition in a much better place than it previously was. Plus, if you include some moderate exercise you will certainly lose at least a pond per week. Good thing about exercise is that if you weight more you will burn more calories.

If you stick to the plan where you will generally lose 1 to 1.5 pounds per week you will probably never again have to deal with so called yo-yo effect, because this is a healthy and sustainable weight loss.

Chapter 2: List and health benefits of Negative Caloric Food

As I previously mentioned food that belongs to the so –called negative caloric food needs to contain a lot of fibers, so vegetable belongs to this group (not all of course), fruits and herbs are also in this group and because of valuable nutrient content that seeds have, you can involve them in smaller amounts maximum 1 teaspoon per meal 2 times a week. From veggies you should include:

Asparagus-it belongs to the healthiest kind of food from ancient times. This plant has been cultivated and used in the Mediterranean kind of cuisine for over 2000 years. Even, Hippocrates, the ancient Greek doctor (known as the father of modern medicine), knew many healthy benefits that asparagus can provide and he used it to treat guts problems such as diarrhea, because asparagus contains high amounts of dietary fibers.

Small asparagus spear contains only 1 kcal and large one 4kcal. Its specific flavor comes from asparagines that are an acidic component which gives this plant its diuretic properties. Also the ratio of some minerals such as potassium and sodium contributes to larger urination. The phytonutrients which asparagus contains acts in a way of anti-inflammatory and anti- cancer processes. Only 3.5 oz or 5 long spears will provide you with all 100% of vitamin K needs that are recommended by Dietary Reference Intakes (DRIs) which are indebted by the Food and Nutrition Board (FNB) at the Institute of Medicine (for adults: women up to 90mcg, men 120mcg on a daily base).   How large of an impact Vitamin K has, you will see through one example, while it acts as an enzyme that is necessary for the creation of proteins needed for proper blood clotting and it plays many more essential roles in our body.

Don't worry, I won't drown you with all beneficial health information for all veggies and fruits that are allowed in this diet; instead I will try to provide some interesting recipes for each ingredient.

Negative caloric asparagus soup

Preparation time/Cook Time: About 20 minutes
Serves: 2
Ingredients:

- 18 oz of asparagus
- 2 cloves of garlic
- 3 cups of water

- salt and pepper
- ¾ a teaspoon of thyme

Preparation:

1. Wash and cut edges of asparagus
2. Put in boiling water and cook until they tender (about 10 minutes). Drain them but leave the broth.
3. Blend asparagus and garlic in fine mixture and return to the saucepan with the asparagus broth, cook for another 10 minutes, and turn off the stove. Add all spices. Serve it with some more grilled asparagus or grilled eggplant complete meal.

Nutrition fact: 56 calories; 0.3g fats; 10.9g carbohydrate;5.4g fibers;5.8 g proteins.

Beetroot belongs to "super food"; this means that it has scientifically proven health benefits for our body. Just one medium sized beetroot (2" dia.) or 3 oz contains only 35 calories, and we all know that you can prepare very tasty salads or smoothies from this delicious veggie.

Red & green smoothie

Ingredients for 1 serve:

- ½ a cup of Mineral Water
- 3.5 oz of beets
- 2 medium sized carrots
- 2 celery sticks
- 1 oz of fresh parsley
- 1 large apple
- 1 scoop of Barley Grass or Alfalfa
- 2 ice cubes.   Mix all

Nutrition fact: 132 calories; 0.9g fats; 30.2g carbohydrate;7.2g fibers;3.2 g proteins.

Broccoli is another low caloric kind of food. The whole "head" contains only 207 calories and one spear just 11 calories, so you can very easily count the amount of calories that you enter. If you prepare it by steaming it then the content of dietary fibers which broccoli contains will better and faster bind with bile acids. The bile is used as an emulsifier for fats and vitamins soluble in oils so in the digestive tract bile acids allows better absorption of fats from the intestine. When you eat sautéed broccoli then you at the same time reduce the possibility of bad cholesterol ending up in your bloodstream in higher amount.

Sautéed Broccoli: Wash and split broccoli flowerets, cut of the stems and cook them over steam or in a saucepan with a very small amount of water. Sautee steams for a few minutes longer than spears, because they are harder so it needs more time for them to tender. Remove from heat, transfer to plate and thus broccoli, with some lemon juice, and then season with salt.

Cabbage- the health benefits of cabbage are numerous, its nutrients help our body to deal with constipation, headaches, stomach ulcers, and with everyday use, very soon our skin becomes cleaner and gets a velvety look, and hair becomes shiny and it thickens. One whole medium sized cabbage (32 oz) contains only 227 calories and one cup of shredded cabbage just 18 calories, so when you chew just one bite or a tablespoon of cabbage your body needs to provide more energy to convert all nutrients from it in an appropriate form so it could be used by our cells. Nevertheless, you must keep in mind that you can't eat it in unlimited quantities, just think of an elephant for example, they also eat just plants but look how big they are, and the main goal of this diet is to lose weight – not to gain it.

Mixed cabbage salad

Preparation time/Cook Time: About 10 minutes
Serves: 1
<u>Ingredients:</u>

- 1 cup of red shredded cabbage
- 1 cup of shredded white cabbage
- ½ a cup of sour beet, sliced
- 1 medium sized chopped raw carrot

Mix all ingredients. Serve as lunch or dinner

<u>Nutrition fact:</u> 97calories; 0.3g fats; 22.6g carbohydrate;6.7g fibers;3.7 g proteins.

Carrots belong to natural cleanser for our body and what is interesting about them is that these veggies are one of the rare kinds of veggies that provide more healthy benefits in cooked form than in raw one. Why? Carrots contain an antioxidant known as lycopen, its amount increases for almost 600 percent when carrots are cooked. Recently it has been proven that low carotenoids levels are the main causes of cardiovascular diseases which can even end with mortal outcomes.

Piquant carrot salad

Preparation time/Cook Time: 5 minutes
Serves: 1

Ingredients:

- 10 oz of carrots
- 4 cloves of garlic
- 3 tbsp. of fresh parsley, finely chopped
- 1 fresh hot Jalapa pepper
- 2 tsp. of dried red sweet paprika spice
- 1 tsp. of ground cumin
- 4 tbsp. of olive oil
- ½ a lemon
- 2 tbsp. of sunflower seeds

Preparation:

1. Cook carrots in a boiling water, but be careful to not overcook them, approximately 5 minutes, drain them and cut into rings.

2. Blend peeled lemon with garlic parsley, pepper, hot pepper and cumin. Add salt to taste. Pour over the carrots combine all and add sunflower seeds and leave in the fridge until serving.

Nutrition fact: 209 calories; 4.3g fats; 42.4g carbohydrate; 11.5g fibers; 6.7 g proteins.

Cauliflower contains substance named sulforaphane that extensively impacts on improving of kidney function. I think that because of this health properties cauliflower needs to be included as much as possible during detoxification phase of negative caloric diet.

Baked cauliflower with mushrooms

Preparation time/Cook Time: 30 minutes
Serves: 4
Ingredients:

- 1 head of cauliflower
- 14 oz of mushrooms
- 4 tbsp. of sesame seeds
- 2 tbsp. of fresh parsley

- 1 tsp. of dill,
- 1 tsp. of basil,
- half a cup of water
- oil for spreading the baking pan, salt, and ground black pepper

Preparation:

1. Preheat the oven to 370°F -190°C
2. Wash the cauliflower; divide it into flowers
3. Cook cauliflower spears in a saucepan in salted water. Drain and set some water aside (half a cup)
4. Cut the mushrooms into thin slices and sauté in a pan until almost water evaporates from them
5. Remove the pan from the heat; add finely chopped parsley, mixed spices, sesame seeds and stir.
6. Line up cauliflower spears in an ovenproof dish, which you previously smeared with a little oil or baking spray, pour over the mixture of mushrooms and bake for about 20 minutes. Serve with some freshly made salad or sliced tomatoes

Nutrition fact: 91 calories; 4.8g fats; 9.1g carbohydrate; 3.8g fibers; 6.1 g proteins.

Celery almost doesn't contain any calories, just one cup contains only 16 kcal and one tablespoon just 1 kcal, so it justifies the title as one of the negative caloric ingredients. In ancient Greek literature, that is older than 1000 years, it was documented that celery was cultivated for medicinal purposes even before 850 B.C. On the other hand ascent Romans didn't eat celery and they believed that celery brings bad luck. Nowadays, we know that celery is an anti-inflammatory kind of grocery, because it contains a high amount of dietary fiber know as pectin. The main role of pectin occurs in the intestine because it binds all harmful substances from our guts and serves as the main ejector when we talk about expelling all toxic substances or any other kind of "trash" that needs to be expelled from the body through the stool, so we could freely say that regular consumption of celery will reduce constipation problems, help our body in detoxification process and so impact on our wellbeing. The stalk of celery is a great source of iron and magnesium and can be eaten raw or in salads, sauces or smoothies. The next recipe is modified Waldorf salad and during the detoxification week you can prepare it as a breakfast meal.

Waldorf salad

Preparation time/Cook Time: 5 minutes

Serves: 1

Ingredients:

- 1 smaller chopped spring of onion,
- Half a sliced peeled sour apple,
- one medium grated celery stalk,
- 1 tbsp. of freshly chopped parsley leaves
- 2 tbsp. of Greek yogurt
- 4 tbsp. of freshly squeezed lemon juice
- 2 chopped walnuts halves

Mix all ingredients and serve.

Nutrition fact: 207 calories; 6.6g fats; 30.8g carbohydrate; 5.7g fibers; 8.9 g proteins.

Cucumber is almost complete made from water and presents one of the best choices of food that will help your body stay hydrated. One large cucumber (10 oz) contains only 34 kcal, and when you cut it into sticks you get a perfect snack. Cucumbers contain one essential nutritive component known as flavonols - antioxidants named fisetin which reduces the risk of developing gastric cancer, especially in women and smokers. Involve cucumber in your meal plan as much as possible, this ingredient is one of the cheapest, its tasty, in can be mixed with any salad, you can add it to many kinds of shakes and smoothies and even use it as a mask for your skin.

Eggplant in cooked form also contains a small amount of calories. One cup only has 35 kcal. Eggplant is actually a fruit like tomatoes, but in everyday environment it is considered as a kind of a vegetable, so that's why I have put it with the list of veggies. Only disadvantage of eggplant is that you shouldn't prepare it too early, because with standing it will start to bitter, so keep in mind that you will get the best taste from eggplant is if you cook it, bake it or roast it shortly before consumption. Here is one proposal for lunch or dinner meal.

Colorful Roasted eggplant

Preparation time/Cook Time: 35 minutes
Serves: 2
Ingredients:

- 1 medium sized eggplant
- 1 medium sized zucchini
- 3 medium sized tomatoes
- 2 yellow peppers
- 1 medium sized onion,
- 2-3 cloves of garlic
- 1 tbsp. of olive oil

- 6 fresh basil leaves
- 6 fresh mint leaves

Preparation:

1. Preheat the oven to 356 °F or 180°C.
2. Wash all vegetables and cut them into 5 mm thick slices.
3. Grease a ceramic container with olive oil and line veggie slices one by one to be compacted. Sprinkle with spices, and cover with aluminum foil or a lid and bake for 30 minutes in the oven.

Nutrition fact: 193 calories; 8.0g fats; 30.2g carbohydrate; 12.7g fibers; 5.9 g proteins.

__Green beans__ or to be more specific 10 pieces (4" long) contain only 17 calories, so a cup of halved beans contains only 34 calories, that's why this veggie belongs to negative caloric food. Even so that color of green beans is obviously green; they contain a valuable content of lutein (beta carotenoids) that most of us link only with red kind of veggies and fruits. This antioxidant protects our vision or eye tissues from sunlight damage. Green beans also contain a specifically kind of flavonoids known as catechins that will help your body reduce body fat from your belly. I need to emphases that these flavonoids also protect prostate, so they should be at your weekly menu at least twice a week.

During the first week on negative caloric diet you should involve **radishes**, **spinach, tomatoes** and **zucchini.**

As from fruits you can freely eat 2 to 3 pieces of apples, apricots, oranges, grapefruits, tangerines , kiwi, pineapples, papaya or 2 to 3 cups of blackberries raspberries, cranberries and strawberries, 1 medium sized cantaloupe, and a quarter of a medium sized watermelon. Fruit is rich with vitamins, antioxidants and you can eat them whole, or prepared in a smoothie. Also you can prepare refreshing lemonade from citrus fruits like lemon or lime and drink it during a day.

Fruits mostly don't have large amount of calories, medium apple for example only has 60 calories and smaller banana goes up to 90 calories, so if you chose mixed fruit salad it average amount of calories should be between 100 and 200 calories.

Nuts should be avoided in higher amounts, but a few halves can be consumed on a daily base. Keep in mind that just 7 walnuts contain 185 calories so always use just a few halves when you add them to your meals.

You can add spices you like, but keep in mind that their taste is best if they are added in small amounts like ¼ of a teaspoon to a teaspoon per meal (depends on what you prepare). In the next chapter I provided you with a list of spices that you can add to your meals.

To manage this more easily here is a proposal of one day meal plan so you could see what kind of food you can prepare during the detoxification week on Negative caloric diet:

A daily meal plan

You will have 5 meals during a day and even so you won't enter the minimum of energy that is needed for basal metabolism which lowest amount is 1200 calories for an adult person, and I need to emphasis that it differs and depends on age, gender, physical activity, but most experts agreed that 1200 calories should present a minimum intake of calories that our body needs.

Note: women who are pregnant or breastfeeding shouldn't adhere to this diet, because they need more nutrients for proper developing of the offspring or if they are breastfeeding for proper production of milk.

For **breakfast** you can consume any smoothies that are made from fresh green leaf veggies combined with tomatoes or cucumber or with some citrus fruits combined with a teaspoon of some seeds like flaxseeds, sesame, and pumpkin, chia or sunflower seeds.

If you don't prefer smoothies you can always make some nice salad spiced with many various kinds of spices. For example, tomatoes go great with oregano or ground nutmeg. What is important is that with much higher consumption of food that contains dietary fibers you won't be hungry during a day, even if you exclude most food that you previously consumed during the first week. Because of fruits that you can consume in higher amounts and which contain natural sugar in a form of fructose you shouldn't have any cravings for some other sweets, but my advice is that before you start with any kind of dieting it would be better if you threw out or gave someone all processed kinds of cookies, sweets and snacks that you have in your house.

Snacks can either be in form of fresh fruits or raw kinds of veggies like sliced carrots or cucumber sticks.

Lunch and **_dinner_** should be prepared from veggies that are cooked, sautéed or roasted, but do not forget that potatoes, legumes and any other kind of fried veggies is strictly forbidden during this first week if you want to properly detoxify your body.

After, this week, which I need to admit is the hardest part of negative caloric diet you can slowly involve other kinds of food such as more dairy products (sour cream, cheese cream, cottage cheese), lean meat (poultry without the skin) and fish such as red fish, cod, tilapia, hake, flatfish, pickerel or any other kind of fish that contains less than 2% of fats. Sardine or anchovy for example, contain almost 5% of fats and salmon, tuna, mackerel and swordfish contain between 5 and 10% of fats so they belong to so-called fatty fish. Start with smaller amounts of meat (3 to 4 oz of meat), you should cut it into smaller cubes or sticks, and prepare them by cooking or roasting them. It's always better to mix meat with some veggies as a salad. For dressing you can use smaller amount of healthy oils like olive oil, use yogurt with some herbs such as oregano, parsley, basil, mint and so on or you can add a handful of nuts instead of classical dressings, because they are after all full of healthy fats in form of omega 3 fatty acids.

Some interesting spices

Do not forget to add some spices, because they will give a better taste to any meal that you prepare. By this I don't mean just salt and pepper, you should also try:

Pimento (Jamaica pepper), is also known as allspice, its taste is sweet, resembles to a mixture of pepper, cloves, nutmeg and cinnamon. You can add this when you marinade meat.

Anise is another sweet spiced kind of herbs that goes great in soups, steaks and risotto. Warm up a handful of whole anise seeds in a pan with a little honey and then pour over yogurt and voile! You will get another refreshing kind of a snack.

Cardamom -you can add it to muesli and you will get a mild sweet and highly aromatic citrus notes meal. When grains are considered you can return it to your everyday meal plan after the third week, but remember just in small amounts. Prepare your own granola and use a tablespoon of it mixed with fresh fruits or a cup of yogurt for breakfast.

Cumin is another good kind of spices which taste reminds me a bit on aromatic walnut-enriched with pepper, a bit pungent that goes great with any kind of fish. Cumin will increase your energy levels in the body, since it contains more iron than any other kind of seasoning.

Kari is in fact a mixture of turmeric, cumin, chili powder, cinnamon and coriander and its taste goes from sweet to very chilly (it depends how much chili powder is added to this mixture).Kari contains a high amount of antioxidants which will reduce the accumulation of fat in the blood vessels, thereby prevents a number of diseases. This spice goes great with eggs or fish.

Saffron gives a distinctive yellowish color to the dishes, and it's one of the most delicious spices, that has a slightly bitter taste. You can add it to soups.

Do not forget to include ginger, garlic, parsley, mint, basil and black pepper in every kind of salad, stewed vegetables and as marinade for meat and fish.

Reminder of food list during each week on the Negative caloric diet

During the first week you will be on fasting mode and you can eat veggies and fruits and in moderate amounts nuts, seeds and yogurt, because your body needs to detoxify. To be sure that you're entering a lower caloric amounts than your body really needs; try not to enter more than 2 pounds of all veggies or fruits that are allowed during this week.

In the second week you can start to re-introduce some other kinds of food like more dairy products, more veggies like sweet potato for example is (stick to one during a day in cooked form). Lean meat and fish are also allowed in small amounts and after that in third week you can increase these amounts a bit.

In third week rice and grains are also allowed, but keep in mind just small amounts as 2 to 3 tablespoons when they are cooked are allowed. This applies to legumes and beans too. Remember, that your goal during Negative caloric diet is to stay below caloric intake that your body really needs so when you re-enter this kind of food always keep the complete recalculation of calories during a day in mind.

Try to keep your breakfast meals less than 400 calories, snacks maximum to 200 calories and lunch and dinner not more than 250 calories and you will stay below 1200 calories during a day. This means that you can eat almost everything for breakfast including even one slice of bread, for snack chose some fruits and for lunch some healthy salad so that you can even eat a smaller steak with sautéed or grilled veggies as side dish for dinner.

Conclusion

Negative caloric diet is not so easy to follow, especially during the first week when most of groceries are restricted to use, but if you are really determined to lose weight and bring your body again in almost perfect condition, then this diet will not fall so hard to you, on the contrary, because the first results are visible only after a few days, I really hope that this will give you the strength to persevere with this dieting regime. The Negative caloric diet is except of the first week, the closest to Mediterranean cuisine where veggies and fruits are present in very high amounts comparing to others kinds of food. The best part of this diet is that you will burn more calories during digestion then you have entered and you will not be hungry during a day because you will enter more dietary fibers that will keep your satiety felling throughout a day. With provided tables of content when veggies are considered I hope that you will be able to combine really tasty kinds of meals, and don't forget to use as much spices as you can in your meals, so you will get more aromatized flavors in this kind of dieting.

Don't forget that:

- Processed food and fast food don't belong to negative caloric diet .

- Avoid soda drinks and any other form of juice in form of factory-produced beverages.

- If you are dinning out than chose restaurants which also have some meals based on vegetarian or vegan kind of cuisine. Always order smaller portion sizes and instead of appetizer chose some healthy salad with no added dressing.

- Even so, that coffee and herbal teas don't contains calories if they are consumed with added sugar in any form then they will be filled with many empty calories, instead of sugar add some spices like cinnamon or drink them without added sugar during the time when you are on negative caloric diet, and of course you need to expel alcoholic beverages during this kind of dieting.

- Real food like veggies and fruits in any kind of form (raw, cooked, sautéed and grilled) belongs to negative caloric food.

- Drink plenty of water, homemade lemonade or juices without added sugar.

- Consume fish, legumes, beans, nuts and meat in moderate amounts and you will be really pleasantly surprised with effects that this diet provides in a very short time.